Canine Mammary Tumor

NIPA® GENX ELECTRONIC RESOURCES & SOLUTIONS P. LTD.
New Delhi-110 034

Canine Mammary Tumor

B.V. Sunil Kumar
Anuradha Sharma
Yashpal Singh Malik
College of Animal Biotechnology
Guru Angad Dev Veterinary and Animal Sciences University
Ludhiana 141004, Punjab, India

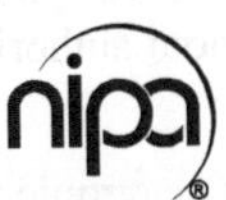

NIPA® GENX ELECTRONIC RESOURCES & SOLUTIONS P. LTD.
New Delhi-110 034

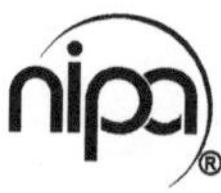

NIPA® GENX ELECTRONIC RESOURCES & SOLUTIONS P. LTD.

101,103, Vikas Surya Plaza, CU Block
L.S.C. Market, Pitam Pura, New Delhi-110 034
Ph : +91 11 27341616, 27341717, 27341718
E-mail: newindiapublishingagency@gmail.com
www: www.nipabooks.com

For customer assistance, please contact
Phone: + 91-11-27 34 17 17
Fax: + 91-11-27 34 16 16
E-Mail: feedbacks@nipabooks.com

ISBN: 978-93-95763-20-2

Manuscript Acquiring Consultant Editor- Dr. Aruna T. Kumar

Editor - Dr. Vrinda Sikri

Composed and Designed by NIPA®.

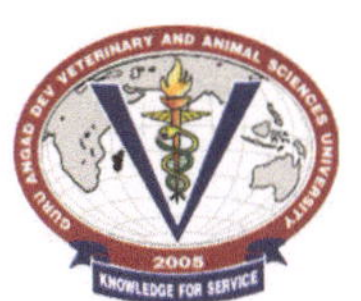

Tel.: 0161-2553360, 2553320
E-mail: vcgadvasu@gmail.com (Official)
inderjeet.dr@gmail.com (Personal)

ਗੁਰੂ ਅੰਗਦ ਦੇਵ ਵੈਟਨਰੀ ਅਤੇ ਐਨੀਮਲ ਸਾਇੰਸਿਜ਼ ਯੂਨੀਵਰਸਿਟੀ
ਲੁਧਿਆਣਾ-141 004, ਪੰਜਾਬ, (ਭਾਰਤ)
GURU ANGAD DEV VETERINARY & ANIMAL SCIENCES UNIVERSITY
LUDHIANA - 141 004, PUNJAB, (INDIA)

ਡਾ. ਇੰਦਰਜੀਤ ਸਿੰਘ
ਉਪ-ਕੁਲਪਤੀ

Dr. Inderjeet Singh
Vice-Chancellor

D.O No
Dated

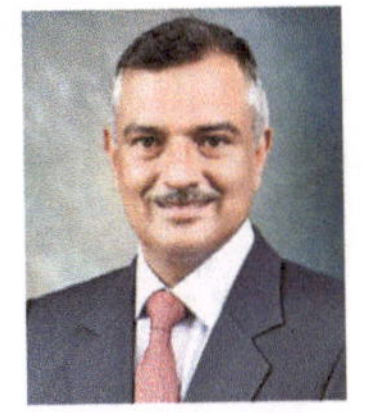

Foreword

Companion animals have become an integral part of our society over the last few decades. Dogs being the most preferred pets need regular checks on their health. Cancer is one among many diseases, having grave prognosis and detrimental effects on canine health. Over the years, canine mammary tumors remain significant cause of death, despite extensive research work in the area. Although survival rates of dogs suffering from localized lesions have been improved significantly, the prognosis for those diagnosed with metastatic tumors still remains poor.

Diagnostics and therapeutics regarding tumors are evolving at a fast pace in recent years. The focus on disease biomarkers, molecular signatures, lifestyles and environments of individual dogs that differentiate their disease susceptibility, treatment responses and prognosis, are the contributing factors to identify patients which are more likely to respond to specific treatments. To achieve these goals, an understanding of tumor biology during its development and progression is needed. In addition, dogs also present as excellent examples for comparative oncology for human breast cancer. Advanced research in dog mammary oncology can serve as references for human mammary oncology and vice-versa. By means of this monograph, an effort has been made to concisely present the established knowledge and latest research about canine mammary tumors.

This monograph 'Canine Mammary Tumor' will serve as a basic information handout for students, clinical veterinary practitioners and researchers. I congratulate the team that has worked in the DBT sponsored project on the 'Development and evaluation of sero-diagnostic assay for timely diagnosis and prognosis of mammary tumors'.

My greetings to all the contributors of this document.

(Inderjeet Singh)

Preface

Canines, as companion and duty/service animals, are highly liked domesticated animals. Therefore, numerous conditions which affect their health needs to be taken care of, for their well-being. Among various fatal conditions which diminish their work potential and shorten their lifespan are tumors and malignancies.

Canine mammary tumor is one such important concern among both owners and Veterinarians. Though frequency of mammary tumors varies in different species, canines are the most frequently affected ones, with prevalence about 3 times higher than humans. Therefore pen side tests and point-of-care diagnostics are to be developed. Treatment regimens and therapeutics are kept up-to-date for efficient management of such conditions.

So, keeping in mind the need of the hour, this monograph on 'Canine Mammary Tumors' has been prepared. This document compiles information on different types of canine mammary tumors and their features, symptoms, their predisposing factors and molecular marker-based diagnosis and prognosis of tumors. It also highlights many other advanced diagnostic techniques and current trends in therapeutics and surgery for their efficient clinical management. Additionally, this monograph lays emphasis on the importance of immunotherapeutics and upcoming and improved vaccines to cure these tumors.

The monograph is worthy, and fully acknowledged to provide the valuable and detailed insight on mammary tumors. Encouragement and support from Dr. J. P. S. Gill, Director of Research and Dr. S.K. Uppal, Dean, Postgraduate Studies, is highly appreciated. Department of Biotechnology, Ministry of Science and Technology, Government of India is also acknowledged for granting funds for research on canine mammary tumors.

We consider that there may be errors and omissions in this piece of work which are requested to be brought into the notice of the authors. It is hoped that this monograph proves useful for veterinary clinicians, students and researchers for their overall awareness and also encourage them to contribute further in the field.

B.V. Sunil Kumar
Anuradha Sharma
Yashpal Singh Malik

Contents

Foreword.......... *v*
Preface.......... *vii*

1. **Introduction**.......... **1**
   - 1.1 Mammary Tumors in Dogs.......... 2
   - 1.2 Mammary Tumors in Other Animals.......... 2
2. **Types of Canine Mammary Tumors**.......... **5**
3. **Classification and Grading**.......... **7**
4. **Canine Mammary Tumor as a Model for Human Breast Cancer**.......... **9**
5. **Incidence**.......... **11**
6. **Predisposing Factors**.......... **13**
   - 6.1 Age.......... 13
   - 6.2 Breed.......... 13
   - 6.3 Hormones.......... 14
   - 6.4 Diet and Obesity.......... 14
   - 6.5 Genetic Factors.......... 15
7. **Signature Markers of Canine Mammary Tumors**.......... **17**
8. **Diagnosis of Canine Mammary Tumors**.......... **19**
   - 8.1 Molecular Diagnosis.......... 19
9. **Treatment and Prognosis**.......... **21**
10. **Modern Therapeutics**.......... **23**
11. **Vaccines**.......... **27**

12. Research Gaps 29

13. Work Done at GADVASU on CMT 33

14. Conclusions 35

15. References 37

16. Index 43

1

Introduction

Canine domestication is an age-old practice which started with guard for humans and other animals, dogs being the favorite companion animals. They have many positive social effects on lives of their owners including enhanced emotional sense and companionship and even reduction of anxiety and mental disorders. Though dogs have proven good for human health, it should be kept in mind that are prone to many disorders and infectious diseases. Healthy life of dogs is attributed to healthy lifestyle, good feeding practices and regular medical care. In addition, an equally important practice is vaccination. Since dogs live in close proximity to human beings and their environment, regular check on their immunity becomes essential, especially when kept as indoor pets. Their illnesses vary from minor issues like dental tartar to fatal diseases like tumors and rabies. Depending upon lifestyle patterns and subsequent body parameters, many predisposing factors increases the susceptibility of dogs to various diseases.

Moreover, inadvertent sniffing and licking by dogs also increases the risk of contracting infections. Common infectious diseases encountered by dogs are infectious canine hepatitis, canine distemper, canine parvoviral diarrhoea, leptospirosis, kennel cough, rabies etc. Due to free wandering, dogs are also susceptible to numerous parasites like haemoprotozoans (babesiosis, ehrlichiosis), heartworms and enteric parasites like ancylostome. Skin disorders are also very common among dogs. Certain pathogens and body conditions like obesity, hormonal imbalances can very commonly lead to tumors and malignancies and the most frequent being canine mammary tumors.

In India core and non-core vaccines are practiced. Core vaccines are given against canine parvovirus, rabies, infectious canine hepatitis, canine distemper while non-core vaccines are given against bordetella and leptospirosis which are region endemicity based. Treatment regimens can easily be followed in dogs which are domesticated and proper care and timely chemotherapy can lead to recovery. Apart from medication, surgical interventions and radiations have proved to be extremely effective in treating certain conditions and disorders. Many advanced diagnostic techniques are employed these days (mechanical/

lab-oriented) detecting molecular markers specific to the diseases leading to sensitive and specific diagnosis.

1.1 Mammary Tumors in Dogs

A neoplasm developing in mammary gland is known as mammary tumor or mammary neoplasia. The frequency of mammary tumor occurrence in different species varies to a great extent. The dog is most affected domestic species, with nearly three times higher prevalence than in human; approximately 50% of all the tumors found in the female dogs are mammary tumors. Mammary tumors are quite rare in goats, cows, mares, sows and ewes. In dogs, mammary tumor (skin neoplasia) is the most common form of tumor found in female dogs and the 2nd most common tumor over all. The risk of mammary tumor development in intact female dog over complete lifespan has been estimated to be about 25%, which is much less (only 1%) in male dogs. Female dogs which are not spayed or which are spayed later than the first heat cycle is more likely to develop mammary tumors (Fig.1). These tumors are often multiple. Obesity at one year of age and eating red meat, increases risk for these tumors as compared to high fat homemade diets.

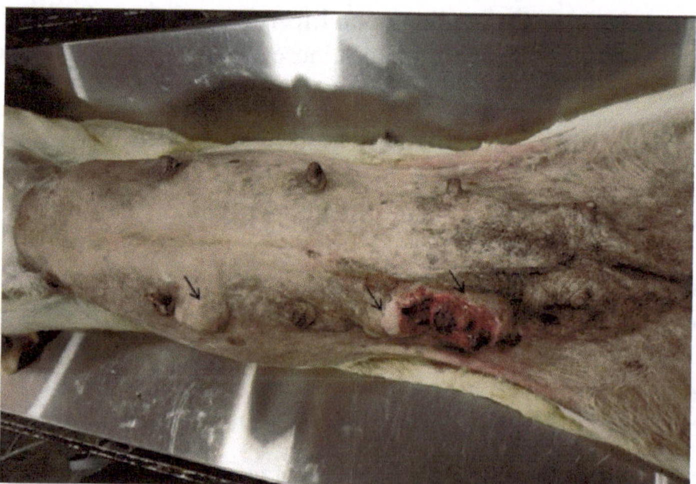

Figure 1: Canine mammary gland tumor

1.2 Mammary Tumors in Other Animals

Mammary neoplasia is the 3rd most common type of neoplasia found in cats, preceded by skin and lymphatic tissue cancers. The risk of mammary tumor incidence gets reduced by 91% in cats which are spayed within six months of their age and by 86% in cats which are spayed within 1st year of their age.

According to the studies, Japanese and Siamese breeds of cats are at higher risk of mammary tumor development and obesity acts as one of the contributing factors. Out of all mammary tumors, up to 80-96% are malignant and mostly adenocarcinomas. Although male cats may rarely develop mammary tumors, and their treatment procedure is similar to that in female cats. Mammary tumors in guinea pigs also occur both in males and females, most of them are benign (a mass of cells or a mild tumor which is not likely to spread), but still 30% are adenocarcinomas. These benign tumors generally do not undergo metastasis, but to prevent recurrence an aggressive surgery is required. Further, majority of mammary tumors in mice are adenocarcinomas, which could be induced by viral infection. Recurrence rates of adenocarcinoma in mice are high, and associated with a poor prognosis.

2

Types of Canine Mammary Tumors

Mammary tumors are either of benign or malignant types. Benign tumors are defined as mass or lump of cells unable to invade the neighboring tissue/ organ and less likely to re-grow after removal. However, malignant tumors are the tumors which have the ability to invade other tissues/ organs and tend to re-grow even after surgical removal. Malignant tumors grow at faster rate as compared to benign tumors. Nearly, 40-50% of canine mammary tumors (CMTs) are malignant.

3

Classification and Grading

CMTs can be classified on the basis of morphologic features, tissue of origin (epithelial, myoepithelial or mesenchymal tissue) or prognosis. The World Health Organization (WHO) classification of canine and feline mammary tumors has categorized CMT into three major categories i) malignant, ii) benign and iii) unclassified tumors. On the basis of histological characteristics, the mammary tumors have been classified into fibroadenomas, adenomas, solid carcinomas (with transformed epithelial cells), tubular adenocarcinomas (with tubule like arrangements), papillary adenocarcinomas (having papillary like projections), anaplastic carcinomas (with highly pleomorphic cells), sarcomas (involvement of connective tissue) and malignant tumors (Fig. 2). Fibroadenomas and adenomas are the types of benign mammary tumors the former contains some connective tissues component in between, and carcinomas, adenocarcinomas and sarcomas come under malignant tumors.

It is very difficult to determine the biological state of tumor by microscopic examination. Once the tumor gets metastasized, it has a poor prognosis, necessitating surgery. Although surgery does not prevent tumor metastasis, the treatment alternatives beyond surgical removal are still limited and have been optimized for different subtypes of CMT.

Also, the early-stage diagnosis of mammary tumors in dogs is very difficult as the signs and symptoms are not very clear. Goldschmidt et al., (2011) has given the criteria for staging of canine mammary tumors (Table 1.) Markers are important tools in its diagnosis. In case of canines, limited research has been done to diagnose the malady at the peripheral blood/serum level. There is a constant search for tumor specific markers that could aid in differential diagnosis of canine mammary neoplasms.

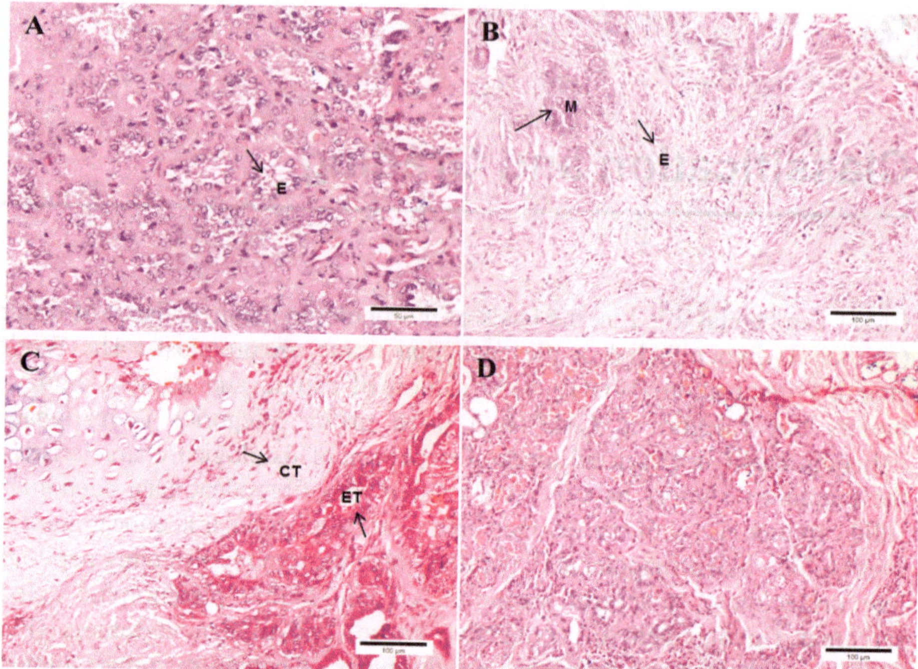

Figure 2: Representative photomicrograph of canine mammary tumors: **(A)** Simple carcinoma showing tubular pattern of the pleomorphic epithelial cells with clear lumen (arrow) (40x), **(B)** Complex carcinoma showing proliferating epithelial cells and myoepithelial cells surrounded by fibrovascular stroma (arrow) (20x), **(C)** Carcinosarcoma/Mixed mammary tumor showing island of pleomorphic epithelial cells along with the presence of cartilage (arrow). (20X), **(D)** Tubulo papillary carcinoma showing islands of pleomorphic epithelial cells surrounded by fibrous stroma (20x) (H&E)

Table 1: Criteria for staging of canine mammary tumors (Goldschmidt et al., 2011)

Stage	Tumor Size	Lymph node Status	Metastasis
I	<3 cm maximum diameter	No involvement of regional lymph node	No distant metastasis
II	3-5 cm maximum diameter	No involvement of regional lymph node	No distant metastasis
III	>5 cm maximum diameter	No involvement of regional lymph node	No distant metastasis
IV	Of any size	Regional lymph node involved	No distant metastasis
V	Of any size	Regional lymph node involved	Distant metastasis

4

Canine Mammary Tumor - as a Model for Human Breast Cancer

Human breast cancer (HBC) is a common malady concomitant with a massive death rate throughout the world. It has been reported that around 1.7 million women are globally identified with breast neoplasia, and out of this, half a million female dies from this terrible disease (Torre et al., 2015). Due to the shocking impacts of breast cancer, prevention, and therapeutic interventions have become a priority-based objective for many researchers to understand the biology of breast cancer disease during its progression and development. But due to the inadequacy of human tissue, the ethical restrictions on conducting experiments on humans require *invitro* and *invivo* models for a better understanding of human breast cancer (Ghoncheh et al., 2016).

A perfect animal model copycats' human disease and regulates the effectiveness of an experimental model to study cancers for risk assessment. Various hormones of the pituitary, ovarian and placental, and the reproductive cycle greatly affect the conversion of the simple normal organ to neoplasm development (Russo, 2015). Numerous species like cats, monkeys, and rodents are being intensely evaluated for this purpose, but none entirely justifies the criteria.

The research on tumors in companion animals constitutes a beneficial and under-utilized resource in cancer research. Moreover, tumors develop in dogs that are usually out-bred, have immunologic competence, and share their living surroundings with human beings. The development of the tumor and its progression is also associated with many interlinked factors between the host environment and the tumor. Therefore, these natural models render a unique perception into cancer biology (Sorenmo et al., 2010; Paoloni & Khanna 2008).

Studies have reported the similarities between CMT and BC, including the prevalence of neoplasm, age, and hormonal etiology. Besides, it also includes similarities in tumor size and invasion of lymph nodes, which directly impacts the clinical outcomes of this disease. Therefore, dogs can be used as a genetic model for studying spontaneous breast cancers (Tabaran & Toma, 2016). Alterations in proteins associated with cell death, cellular proliferation, and differentiation in HBC and CMT corroborate the use of the canine model to comprehend the molecular pathways tangled in mammary gland carcinogenesis (Kumaraguruparan et al., 2006).

5

Incidence

The incidence of mammary tumor accounts for 25% of all the recorded tumors in dogs worldwide. Overall, about 198 cases of CMT are recorded per one lakh female dogs annually throughout the world which is quite an alarming percentage (Gray et al., 2020). Malignancy has also been recorded up to 45% which increases the fatality among morbid cases.

Epidemiology of CMT is poorly documented particularly in India. In an epidemiological study conducted on canine tumors in Jammu in 2018, the overall prevalence was only 2% over a period of one year. The malignant tumors accounted 41.66% of the mammary tumors (Sharma et al., 2018). The rate of benign and malignant tumors incidence was reported as 46% and 54%, respectively. In another study conducted on the incidence of CMT in Ludhiana (Punjab) in 2020, it was found that 33.96% tumors were benign and 66.03% were malignant (Dash et al., 2020).

Another study carried out on canine mammary neoplasms in Puducherry, India in 2018; concluding 77 cases (0.67%) out of 11,423 reported canine cases which were affected with neoplasia of mammary gland (Nadhiya et al., 2018). Majority of the cases belonged to intact dogs (92%) compared to spayed ones (8%). In a different study in Gujarat in 2010, it was found that out of 2070 canine cases, 158 (7.63%) were found to have neoplastic conditions and amongst them 63 cases (39.87%) were of CMT. Therefore, the overall occurrence of CMT was 0.75% of total canine cases (Dhami et al., 2010). Another study from Punjab in 2012 examined 139 canine biopsy samples and on the basis of histopathology, 109 samples were found to be neoplastic and 60 samples were non-neoplastic. Out of 109 neoplastic biopsy samples, 51 were CMT and 58 were other tumors (Gupta et al., 2012). In a study conducted to assess the occurrence of canine neoplasia in Bareilly, Utter Pradesh, among 403 cases, 42.93% cases of canine transmissible venereal tumor (CTVT) were recorded followed by mammary gland tumors (33.50%) and skin and other tumors (23.57%). In general, more cases of mammary neoplasia were recorded in females than that in males. However, in case of skin and other tumors more cases were recorded in males than in females (Khimta et al. 2011).

A similar study has been conducted in the Veterinary University of Himachal Pradesh, India, during the period from 2006 to 2008. It was reported that incidence of mammary tumor, genital tumors and other tumors comprising skin and bone tumors in dogs were 13.33%, 33.33%, 53.33% respectively, (Umeshwori et al. 2011).

6

Predisposing Factors

6.1 Age

Age is one of the most important risk factors for developing mammary tumors in dogs. A comprehensive study carried on dogs has found that the risk of mammary tumors become significant by 8 years of age and increases linearly thereafter. The age of onset of tumors, however, may vary depending on the life span of the dog breed. An average age of CMT onset is 8-11 years, indicating as a condition of the middle-aged or older dogs. Mammary tumors are generally rare in dogs under 3 years of age, unless the dogs have been given exogenous hormones such as progestins.

6.2 Breed

Most consistently listed breeds in which mammary tumor occur include, English springer spaniel, Brittany, Cocker spaniel, English setter, Pointer, Afghan hound and German shepherd, in addition to the smaller breeds such as Poodle, Maltese, Chihuahua, Beagle, Dachshund and Terriers. These studies clearly show that the risk for mammary tumors has some breed association and, therefore, having a genetic component. Pure breeds of dogs are generally at a greater risk i.e., known to account for 80% of the submitted cases. Some studies have further shown that certain lines within specific breeds are at more risk than others.

Samoyed breed was found to be most commonly suffered from canine mammary tumors (34.10%) followed by Doberman (19.65%) German Shepherd (9.83%) non-descript (8.10%), Labrador Retriever (7.57%) Pointer (5.78%) Crossbred (5.20%), Dachshund (2.89%), Boxer (2.31%), Cocker Spaniel (1.73%), Lhasa Apso (1.16%) and Tibetan Mastiff, Poodle and Irish Setter breeds (0.58% each). In Indian scenario, various scientists have recorded in common a highest incidence of canine mammary tumors for Spitz breed.

6.3 Hormones

Early life exposure to endogenous ovarian hormones is an important source and cause of mammary tumor development in dogs. The risk for developing mammary tumor in dogs decreases significantly when spayed prior to their first estrus, incidence is only 0.5% as compared to intact female dogs and between the first and second estrus, incidence is 8%. With the advancement of spaying age, the incidence of tumors also increases (26% between the second and fourth estrus) and no positive effect of spaying has been found after the fourth estrus. However, some subsequent studies have shown that later spaying may provide some protection. A study by Sonnenschein and colleagues (1991) documented that significant protection is associated with spaying prior to the fourth estrus cycle and between the 4th and 6th estrus cycle. The protective effect from ovarian hormone suppression is highly dependent on dose. The effect is clearly higher in patients with minimal to no exposure and reduces relatively faster after the first few years.

Other reproductive factors including irregularity of estrus cycle, pseudo-pregnancy, and pregnancy which may cause physiological changes in endogenous levels of hormones, do not significantly influence the risk of mammary tumor development in dogs. Thus, an exposure to ovarian hormones in the first two estrus cycles poses the highest risk and exogenous exposure or pharmacological supply of both estrogen and progestin hormones further potentiates the risk for mammary tumors development.

6.4 Diet and Obesity

A large case-control study by Sonnenschein and colleagues (1991) investigated the association between diet, body conformation and risk for developing mammary tumors and observed a significantly decreased risk in dogs that were thin at 9-12 months of age when compared with the control dogs. In a study, dogs which were fed red meat and the dogs which developed obesity at one year of age developed mammary tumors, indicating a correlation between diet and mammary cancer. Obesity is considered to add up in breast cancer risk in women after menopause by increasing circulating estrogen and production of local estrogen by aromatases. It is possible that obesity increases the risk for development of mammary tumors in canines through similar mechanisms.

In a study a dietary questionnaire was used to assess macronutrient intake along with the measurement of the fatty acid composition of subcutaneous adipose tissue and the plasma concentrations of retinol and selenium. In which they found that the intake of homemade meals (compared to that of commercial foods) were significantly related to a higher incidence of tumors and dysplasia. Mammary tumor risk was found to be positively associated with the intake of red meat and negatively with the intake of poultry meat.

6.5. Genetic Factors

Along with hormones, genetic predisposition also plays a role in developing mammary gland tumors. Inactive tumor suppressor genes, translocation, point mutations, and oncogene amplifications are among the genetic changes identified in human breast cancer. Oncogenes and their receptors coded by growth factors have been found to overexpress in relation to the uncontrolled growth of the tumor (Misdorp, 1988). The greater susceptibility of a breed to mammary tumor occurrence can also be traced back to its genetic makeup.

Some genes dominate the risk of developing mammary tumors, though reports conclude certain families are more prone to breast cancer which results in the prediction of genetic predisposition of breast cancer (Rivera & Euler, 2011).

In the past, researchers have observed BRCA1, a breast cancer susceptibility gene on chromosome no. 17, using the positional cloning method (Miki et al., 1994). BRCA2 was localized on chromosome 13 through linkage analysis (Wooster et al., 1994). BRCA1 & BRCA2 together act as tumor suppressor genes; hence the inherited mutation in the BRCA1 and BRCA2 genes in women are found to cause breast cancer (Rivera et al., 2009). The breast cancer susceptibility genes are grouped according to their risk development, i.e., high, intermediate, or low risk (Ripperger et al., 2009). Some genes contribute to the highest risk of breast cancer in women viz. checkpoint kinase 2 (CHEK2), fibroblast growth factor receptor 2 (FGFR2), transformation-related protein (TP53), phosphate and tensin homolog (PTEN) (Walsh et al., 2006). These genes are involved in the differentiation of cells, proliferation and cause tumor suppression. The intermediate gene groups include ataxia-telangiectasia mutated kinase (ATM), CHEK2, BRCA1 interacting protein C-terminal kinase (BRIP1), RAD50 homolog. The least risk development gene group in breast cancer includes FGFR2, lymphocyte-specific protein (LSP1), mitogen-activated protein kinase (MAP3K1), and thymocyte selection associated high mobility group box (TOX). Around 10 human breast, cancer-associated genes have been studied with respect to charcot-marie-tooth (CMT) incidence. Among them, matrix metalloproteinase 11, 3 and their inhibitors have been found to be associated with CMT occurrence (Pandey et al., 2017; Kaur et al., 2016; Kumar & Kataria, 2013). A point mutation in BRCA1 and BRCA2 genes in canines has been associated with CMT incidence (Ochiai et al., 2001). RAD51 is a DNA-repairing protein that has been shown to mediate

CMT occurrence (Kato et al., 2000). RAD51 gene has been reported to be overexpressed in 80% lymph node metastasis, and upregulation of this gene in CMT was confirmed by qRT-PCR analysis (Klopfleisch & Gruber, 2009 A). Among the heat shock proteins (HSP), serum HSP90 level has been found to increase in CMT subjects (Kumar et al., 2018). Another breast cancer-associated gene, mammaglobin B, has also been found to be upregulated in CMT (Pandey et al., 2015; Pandey et al., 2018). Tissue level expression of mammaglobin B has been studied in CMTs by immunohistochemistry and is found to be upregulated in CMT tissues (Pandey et al., 2018).

7

Signature Markers of Canine Mammary Tumors

There are countless biomarkers present in cells related to and determining the progress of a disease. Identifying these markers could aid in detecting cells with metastatic potential (Ramaswamy et al., 2003).

The elevation of cyclo-oxygenase (Cox-2) expression was observed in CMT cases through enzyme immunoassay (Queiroga et al., 2005). In further study, enhanced expression of BRAC1and BRAC2 genes, certain enzymes such as matrix metalloproteinases (MMP-2 and MMP-9) by immunohistochemical examinations, and Bcl-2 & Bcl-XL elevated level in dogs with mammary neoplasm have been reported by Queiroga et al. (2011b).

In recent studies, overexpression of ki-67 nuclear nonhistone protein, proliferating cell nuclear antigen (PCNA)-auxiliary DNA polymerase δ and p53 tumor suppresser gene at the onset of the canine mammary tumors was reported by Kaszak et al. (2018). Reports advocate the up-regulation of certain heat shock proteins such as HSP70 (Badowska-Kozakiewicz& Malicka, 2012), HSP90B1 (Kumar et al., 2018), and HSP27 (Birdi et al., 2019) in mammary tumors of dogs. Various oncogenes viz. c-myc, Cyclin A, erbB2, FIS1, IL3, int-1/wnt-1, RAS have also been associated with CMT progression (Pawaiya et al. 2011).

The expression of Alcohol dehydrogenase 1 (ALDH1), a cytosolic enzyme responsible for oxidizing intracellular aldehydes involved in early stem cell differentiation has been found to increase in various CMT histotypes indicating poor prognosis. In a study on 24 cases of CMT, it was detected that 83% of the cases have increased expression of ALDH1 and it was observed in benign lesions, invasive cells and cells undergoing epithelial to mesenchymal transition (EMT) i.e., all types of tumors. Increased expression of ALDH1 indicates its role in EMT. Its activity helps cells in switching of cell from one type to another which is the property of the stem cells so its level is found to be increased in tumor cells as well. The expression of ALDH1 was evident in invasive cells in cases of carcinoma and carcinosarcoma. It indicated possible role of ALDH1 in invasion and tumor progression from benign to invasive (Savagner 2010 and Gavhane et al. 2016).

8

Diagnosis of Canine Mammary Tumors

A thorough history with complete physical examination including careful palpation of the mammary glands should be performed. As there are chances that dogs may be suffering from any other systemic ailments during middle to old age. In dogs with multiple tumors, all tumors should be excised and their location and size should be noted. Histopathological examination of the excised tumors should be carried out to classify mammary gland tumors. Mammary tumors are classified based on some of the parameters i.e., tumor size, lymph nodes, metastasis. Therefore, to stage a dog with mammary tumors information of these parameters needs to be collected and recorded. If lymph nodes are palpable and/or clinically enlarged, fine-needle aspiration should be performed for cytological evaluation. The technique is less invasive but with higher accuracy. Thoracic radiographs remain the mainstay for diagnosing the metastatic condition. The mammary tumors most commonly metastasize into lungs in dogs. The staging of CMTs becomes necessary as it is likely to confer some prognostic significance and provide guidance to veterinarians to make treatment decisions.

8.1 Molecular Diagnosis

Immuno-phenotyping, taking the advantage of distinct immune profiles of normal human breast cells and canine mammary cells, is used for the diagnosis of mammary tumors and for targeting treatment therapies. Type I acidic cyto-keratins (CKs) 18,19 and Type II basic cyto-keratins are the characteristic markers of luminal epithelial cells whereas myoepithelial cells are characterized by Type I acidic 14, 17 CKs and Type II basic 5 and 6 CKs. Myoepithelial cells in CMTs are more proliferative than human breast cancers and also express various markers like calponin, p63, smooth muscle actin, vimentin, P-cadherin, epidermal growth factor receptor, CD10, 14-3-3 sigma protein and napsin A.

For molecular classification of human breast cancer and prediction of the possible treatment immunohistochemistry (IHC) is routinely used. Due to existing time and cost constraints, even after considerable efforts in the field of molecular diagnosis over past years, we are still largely dependent on IHC assessment of different markers like human epidermal growth factor receptor (HER-2), progesterone receptors, estrogen receptors, Ki-67 etc. for breast cancer classification. Despite of well-established IHC based classification and diagnosis in human breast cancer, results obtained in CMTs are highly variable and even contradictory, which results in enormous difference in molecular subtypes of CMTs among different investigators.

9

Treatment and Prognosis

Surgical removal is the routine treatment method for mammary tumors, however, there is no consensus on the optimal procedure. There are supporting factors for every surgical procedure conducted for mammary tumors including lumpectomy (removal of tumor only), mastectomy (affected gland removal only), radical mastectomy (complete mammary gland and associated lymphatic tissue removal) and modified radical mastectomy (removal of complete mammary gland, lymph nodes and associated chest muscles).The more extensive procedures do not increase survival in dogs when compared to the other procedures, and the benefits of the simpler procedures are clear. Further, the radical mastectomy increases the disease-free interval but not the survival duration in cats.

In theory, the use of anticancer medications for treatment of micro-metastatic illness, adjuvant chemotherapy is considered as a rational treatment option. However, chemotherapy has not been approved as a promising treatment option for CMTs. The fact that approximately only a half of the CMTs which are identified as malignant on histopathologic examinations actually behaves that way, adds to the complexity of measuring the response to adjuvant chemotherapy. On several types of malignant tumors, COX inhibitors (e.g., deracoxib) have been found to exhibit anti-angiogenic and anti-cancer properties. Doxorubicin and deracoxib combination have exhibited synergistic effect on breast cancer cells invitro. Deracoxib potentiates the apoptosis induction by increasing the doxorubicin mediated in cell cycle progression at G0/G1 and enhances the anti-proliferative potential of doxorubicin by modulating expression of B-cell leukemia/lymphoma 2 (Bcl-2) protein.

Clinical trials are required to assess whether the synergistic effect of doxorubicin and deracoxib could provide us an effective and viable clinical treatment strategy for CMTs at a relatively lower dose and less side effects as compared to treatment with doxorubicin alone. In cats, the combination of drugs cyclophosphamide and doxorubicin has been tested for mammary tumor treatment but its efficacy was limited. The clinical efficacy of other treatment methods like anti-estrogenic compounds and radiation therapy is also not concluded up to the mark.

The treatment with nonsteroidal anti-inflammatory drug (NSAID) piroxicam has shown promising outcome against canine inflammatory mammary carcinoma, which is a subtype of mammary tumor and difficult to treat either surgically or medically. This outcome is in line with the current need of a metronomic low-dose treatment therapy with anti-angiogenic and anti-cancer effects against various malignancies. Above discussed treatment strategies for CMTs are summarized in Fig. 3.

The prognosis is based on multiple factors. In dogs, most mammary tumors which are lethal are going to cause death within 1 year. Sarcomas are associated with shorter survival times than carcinomas. Other factors viz. tumor size, nuclear differentiation and involvement of lymph nodes, also affect the prognosis. In cats, tumor size is important; cats with tumors >3 cm in diameter have a median survival time of 6 months, but cats with tumors <2 cm in diameter have a median survival time of >4 years.

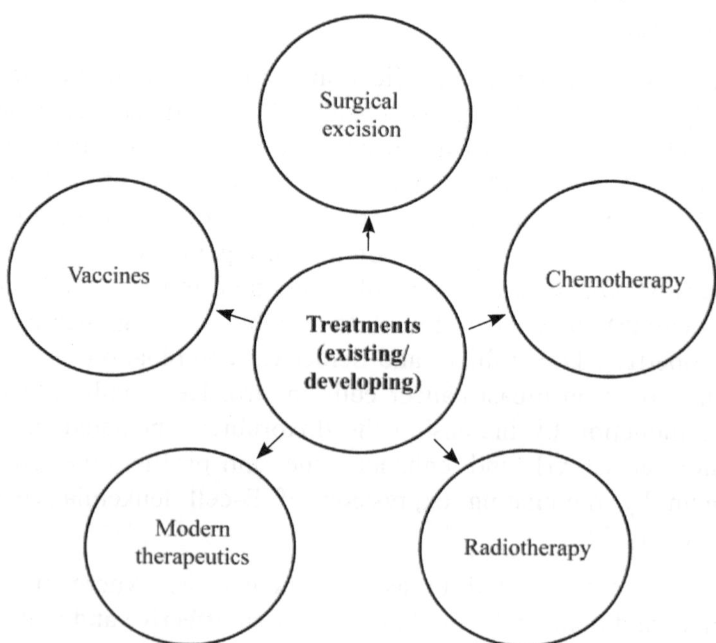

Figure 3. Different type of existing and developing treatment strategies for CMTs

10

Modern Therapeutics

In addition to the conventional treatment methods i.e., surgery, chemotherapy and radiotherapy, there are some adjuvant targeted therapies which block the growth of cancer by altering the individually expressed specific molecules responsible for tumor cell proliferation, survival, metastasis or microenvironment. The majorly studied adjuvant therapies include use of hormones, tyrosine kinase receptors, anti-cyclooxygenases, anti-tumor suppressor gene p53 and epithelial-mesenchymal transition inhibition.

The main aim of hormonal therapy (Table 2) is to inhibit the hormone induced stimulation of carcinoma cells, which could be achieved either by ovariohysterectomy or different treatments like use of specific estrogen receptor modulators (SERMS), aromatase inhibitors for suppression of estrogen synthesis etc. A commonly used estrogen receptor (ER) antagonist drug tamoxifen for treatment of ER positive breast cancer in women, has also been tested against CMTs. However, it is not a viable treatment option in dogs due to associated side effects. Ovariohysterectomy is considered as a better and practical solution. The use of hormonal therapy in CMTs is based on the evidence of hormone dependency of these tumors as well as lessons learnt from hormonal therapy outcomes from human breast cancer. This therapy significantly ameliorates the recurrence of breast cancers and prolongs the survival rates in women having breast cancers positive for hormone receptors. However, the results of the canine investigations, which are all retrospective and non-randomized, are contradictory. Detailed research and prospective randomized trials, where effect of OHE is studied in context of hormone receptor status, are required to determine the role of hormonal therapy in CMTs.

Modern era drugs are majorly targeted to p53 gene and bcl-2 proteins to cure the cancer in dogs. But they have side effects due to alteration in genes. Hence the need is of gene therapy-based drugs which directly kills cancer cells and has oncolytic property. One of that gene is VP3 gene of chicken infectious anemia virus which was considered as alternative option of treatment for CMT. Oncolytic potential of recombinant VP3 of chicken infectious anemia virus was established in CMT by DNA fragmentation using ladder pattern/ agarose gel electrophoresis assay and Terminal deoxynucleotidyl transferase dUTP nick end labeling (TUNEL) assay.

It has been found that initially virus utilizes mitochondria mediated pathway to kill the cells followed by death receptors and endoplasmic reticulum mediated mechanism at later stages. It has also been observed that theVP3 protein obtained from Indian isolate of Canine adenovirus (CAV) can induce cell death among tumor cells of canine origin in vitro. The extent of regression by VP3 gene in this study was 11.9%. Most of the expression of VP3 protein takes place in nucleus where it aggregated in fine granular pattern in CMT cells (Pandey et al., 2012).

In a comparative study to check the effectiveness of cinnoline sulfonamide therapeutic drug in CMT and Venereal tumors, the chemotherapeutic agent administered @ 500 mg orally was found very much effective to treat both mammary tumor (66%) and venereal tumor (50%) cases. The drug was effective in small size (2-3 cm) and recently developed tumors. The side effects were found to be temporary and minimal (Saxena et al. 2011)

It has been reported that NS1 gene of canine parvovirus @ 200 μg intra-tumoral injections at weekly intervals up to 4 weeks has proved success to treat 10 CMT subjects. The treatment led to significant shrinkage of the tumors in 4 weeks. It was also observed that as the tumor regression took place, the increased vascular connective tissue is seen from engorged blood vessels in the fibrous connective tissues with few alveolar packets. The spaces surrounded by fibrous connective tissues are indicative of wearing off of regressed tumor masses (Verma et al. 2014).

Tyrosine kinase receptors (Table 2) catalyze various phosphorylation reactions of target proteins that are involved in cellular metabolism, proliferation, migration, survival and apoptosis as well as neovascularization by epithelial cell activation. Tyro-kinase inhibitors (TKIs) are considered as biotechnological breakthroughs in breast cancer treatment. TKIs are differentiated from other drugs with a suffix "nib" placed at the end of generic name. Among Tyrosine kinase receptors, colony stimulating factor 1 (CSF-1), HER-2, stem cell factor /c-Kit Receptor, platelet-derived growth factor receptors (PDGFRs), and vascular endothelial growth factor receptors (VEGFRs), are constitutively activated or overexpressed in human and canine tumors. These TKIs target extracellular or intracellular proteins, inhibit ATP binding (competitive inhibition) and subsequent phosphorylation events, impeding the signal transduction to the nucleus, thus disrupting the process of cellular proliferation and differentiation. The majority of TKIs are administered orally, which benefits animal welfare by reducing stressful conditions and making administration easier for the owner. Several attempts to inhibit these receptors have been made in veterinary oncology. Some TKIs used in human oncology have diverse activities depending on the receptors inhibited (e.g., Sunitinib inhibits c-KitR, colony-stimulating factor (CSF-2), Platelet-derived growth factor receptor (PDGFR), and Vascular endothelial growth factor receptor (VEGFR) and can be used to treat a different cancer.

In carcinogenesis, the tumor suppressor gene p53 plays a crucial role. After tetramerization, the p53 protein limits cell proliferation and induces cell cycle arrest. Since the mutations in the p53 gene have such a large impact on cancer growth, researchers are working hard to figure out mechanisms to block this effect. In CMT cells, there has only been one investigation on p53 treatment which studied the effect of exportin-1 overexpression. By overexpressing exportin-1, neoplastic cells can boost nuclear p53's cytoplasmic translocation, blocking its DNA binding and anti-proliferative activity. The addition of KPT-185 and KPT-355 designed compounds that block exportin-1, decreased proliferation, promoted the cell cycle arrest and apoptosis in CMT cells in vitro.

The epithelial–mesenchymal transition (EMT) is a complicated process in which epithelial cells lose their traits and take on mesenchymal characteristics. It is required for various embryonic stages and organ development, neoplastic infiltration, metastasis, cell migration and wound healing. Epithelial cells get detached and acquire motility as well as invasiveness through the extracellular matrix, allowing them to eventually penetrate blood and lymphatic vessels and to colonize various organs. A variety of pharmacological drug candidates have been developed to target EMT in CMTs, including melatonin, artemisinin, metformin, simvastatin and others.

Table 2: Types of modern adjuvant targeted therapeutics for mammary tumors

S. No.	Type of Adjuvant targeted therapy	Targets	Drug molecules/candidates
1.	Hormonal Therapy	Estrogen, progesterone, growth hormone, prolactin, melatonin, aromatase and their receptors etc.	Estrogen inhibitors (Tamoxifen, Indole-3-carbinol), aromatase inhibitors (letrozole, flutamide), progesterone inhibitors (megestrol acetate, medroxyprogesterone acetate, mifepristone, onaprestone), melatonin and prolactin receptor inhibitors
2.	Tyrosine kinase receptors	HER-2 VEGF family c-Kit	Anti-HER2 agents (trastuzumab, pertuzumab, lapatinib, neratinib, afatinib, trastuzumabemtansine) Anti-VEGF (or anti-angiogenesis) agents (bevacizumab, pazopanib, sunitinib, sorafenib) Anti-c-Kit agents (Masitinib, toceranib
3.	Antitumor gene suppressor p53	Exportin-1	Exportin inhibitors (KPT-185, KPT-355)
4.	Anti-cyclooxygenases	COX-1, COX-2, COX-3	Non-steroidal anti-inflammatory drugs (NSAIDs- meloxicam, piroxicam) and COX inhibitors (Coxibs- firocoxib, deracoxib, cimicoxib, robenacoxib, mavacoxib)
5.	Epithelial-Mesenchymal transition inhibition	Cadherins	Cadherin inhibitors/ targeting agents (Metformin, simvastatin, artemisinin)

11

Vaccines

One of the most promising areas of veterinary research these days is cancer immunotherapy and the development of CMT vaccines. DNA vaccines, also known as gene vaccines, are designed to transfer functional genes to target cells, allowing them to express functional proteins. Because endonucleases may easily access bare DNA, it requires a reliable and safe delivery route, which might be biological or non-biological. Different delivery strategies have been tried in human breast tumors to transport tumor antigens such Mucin-1 (MUC-1), Twist, HER-2, mammaglobin-1 and p53, as well as immunostimulatory molecules like IL-12 and IL-6. There have been various studies/ trials in canine animals using different molecules like IL-12, HER-2 and IFN-γ as vaccine candidates, with no clinically relevant outcomes or long-lasting cell mediated and humoral immune response outcomes.

A p62 based DNA vaccine with anticancer potential was studied in mice with CMT xenografts and dogs having mammary tumors. P62 is a protein essential for selective macro-autophagy that is dispensable for majority of tissues but crucial for development and persistence of tumors. This vaccine when administered intramuscularly exhibited a partial response without any significant secondary effects. Its anti-tumoral effects were related to lymphocyte infiltration and tumor encapsulation.

11

12

Research Gaps

Although there have been multiple biomarkers for mammary tumors both in human and canines reported over the time (Table 3), but no absolute biomarker for diagnosis and prognosis of CMT has been found yet. Out of several studies on clinical applications of different mammary tumor biomarkers, some showed a particular promising biomarker, on the other hand controversial results also existed for the same. For example, HER-2, which is one of the most prominent bio-marker both in HBC and CMT. HER-2 overexpression is associated with poor prognosis and reduced overall survival of the subject, but there are studies available which suggest no difference in HER-2 expression between benign and malignant tumors and studies showing HER-2 expression suggesting prolonged survival (Kaszak et al., 2018). Various biomarkers of mammary tumors are not mammary tumor specific such as p53, COX-2, PCNA etc. These markers undergo alterations in their expression level in all tumors. By keeping this in mind we need to device a panel of different markers to ensure the correct prognosis and diagnosis of canine mammary tumors. There are limited studies and only few commercial kits (for human) available using such combinations (Table 4).

Further, early detection of tumor onset is still a target to achieve. Most of the established mammary tumor biomarkers are detectable in later stages of tumors which reduce the chances of successful treatment and prolonged survival. Although CA 15-3 (Mucin-1) is considered specific and very good marker for HBC and CMT detection and prognosis, but available studies are not sufficient for veterinary patients.

In terms of treatment, the already existing treatment strategies such as surgery, radiotherapy, chemotherapy and non-steroidal inflammatory drugs (NSAID) are associated with various side effects such as chances of recurrence of tumors, increased chances of catching infections, prolonged healing period for injuries or infection, loss of appetite etc. Hence selection of suitable treatment strategy, particularly for pets is a big dilemma. Researchers are making attempts to device gene-targeted, tumor specific treatment therapies and therapeutic vaccines to bring out more fruitful result, possibly with least side effects,. Though more such studies are required to be conducted in future.

Table 3: Biomarkers for canine/ human mammary tumors

S. No.	Marker	Expression	Dog/Human	Reference
Apoptosis and Cancer cell proliferation				
1.	Ki-67	Enhanced expression in mammary tumor, detected using IHC and ELISA, used to determine tumor subtype along with other tumor markers	Dog, human	Nowak et al. (2015); Kaszak et al. (2018)
2.	Proliferating cell nuclear antigen (PCNA)	Proliferation biomarker, used for breast cancer evaluation along with other markers like ER, PR, Ki-67 or HER-2	Dog, human	Jurikova et al. (2016); Kandefer-Gola et al. (2016); Kaszak et al. (2018)
3.	p53	Biomarker for cell neoplastic transformation, apoptosis and cell division, high expression is associated with poor prognosis	Dog, human	Klopfleisch et al. (2009); Pan et al. (2017); Kaszak et al. (2018)
Biomarkers for metastasis				
4.	E-Cadherin	Downregulation/ loss of E-cadherin expression related to epithelial-mesenchymal transition, cell migration, metastasis and tumor aggressiveness	Dog, human	Li et al. (2017); Nowak et al. (2015); Kaszak et al. (2018)
5.	Glycoprotein CEA	CEA overexpression in tumors as compared to healthy subjects, biomarker for early detection of recurrence and metastasis	Dog, human	Campos et al. (2012); Di Gioia et al. (2016); Kaszak et al. (2018)
6.	CA 15-3 (Mucin-1)	Overexpression in mammary carcinomas	Dog, human	Manauli et al. (2012)
Biomarkers for Angiogenesis				
7.	VEGF	Higher expression is associated with poor prognosis of HBC and CMT	Dog, human	Queiroga et al. (2011); Zajkowska et al. (2016)
8.	EGFR (HER-1)	Higher expression is associated with increased angiogenesis, tumor size and poor prognosis	Dog, human	Carvalho et al. (2013)

9.	HER-2	Higher expression of HER-2, poorer the prognosis and survival	Dog, human	De Pedro et al. (2015), Campos et al. (2015)
Hormone receptors				
10.	Estrogen receptor (ER), Prolactin receptor (PR)	Expression of ER and PR is related to favorable prognosis	Dog, human	Kaszak et al. (2018)
Biomarkers of Inflammation				
11.	COX-2	Higher COX-2 expression is associated with tumor recurrence and malignancy	Dog, human	Hugo et al. (2015); Queiroga et al. (2010)
Other Markers				
12.	BRCA-1 and BRCA-2 mutations	BRCA-1 mutation (loss of expression) associated with malignant tumors, however, the role BRCA-2 mutation is controversial	Dog, human	Kaszak et al. (2018)
13.	MiRNA	Different miRNAs act as diagnostic and prognostic markers in CMT and HBC	Dog, human	Kaszak et al. (2018)
14.	Collagen Fiber Imaging (Number and length)	More aggressive tumor, smaller the size of collagen fibers	Dog	Gracia et al. (2021)
15.	Circulating cell free DNA (cf-DNA)	Higher concentration and higher integrity index of short and long fragments of-cfDNA in neoplastic subjects than non-neoplastic and healthy subjects	Dog, human	Beffagna et al. (2017), Agostini et al. (2012)
16.	Cancer Stem Cells (CSCs)	CD44+/CD24– phenotype of CSCs is associated with high-grade CMT and poor prognosis in HBC	Dog, human	Im et al. (2015)
17.	Circulating Tumor cells	Acts as biomarkers of metastatic potential, play role in disease monitoring	Dog, human	Kaszak et al. (2018)

18.	Heat shock protein-27 (HSP-27)	Elevated HSP-27 levels in CMT, antibodies to HSP-27 in HBC are associated with improved survival	Dog, human	Birdi et al. (2019), Cornoy et al. (1998)

Table 4: Some Commercial kits/assays for mammary tumor detection

S. no.	Commercial Kit description	Marker accessed	Reference
1.	Dual-probe FISH assay PathVysion (Abbott France SAS, Rungis, France)	HER-2	Cayre et al. (2007)
2.	probe pharmDx (Dako France SAS, Trappes, France)	HER-2	Cayre et al. (2007)
3.	mono-probe INFORM (Ventana Medical Systems SA, Illkirch, France) FISH assays	HER-2	Cayre et al. (2007)
4.	CISH assay SPoT-Light (Zymed Laboratories Inc., San Francisco, CA, USA)	HER-2	Cayre et al. (2007)
5.	Xpert® Breast Cancer STRAT4 (Cepheid, Sunnyvale, CA, USA)	ESR1/PGR/ ERBB2/MKi67 mRNA	www.cepheid.com
6.	Aware BREAST SELF-EXAMINATION kit (NiN Healthcare, Newport beach, CA, USA)	Sense based breast self-exam	ninhealthcare.com
7.	Multiplexed Autoantibody Signature for Serological Detection of Canine Mammary Tumors (developed, not commercialized yet)	TPI, PGAM1, MNSOD, CMYC & MUC1	Hussain et al. (2018)

13

Work Done at GADVASU on CMT

In GADVASU, under the DBT sponsored project on "Development and evaluation of serodiagnostic assay for timely diagnosis and prognosis of mammary tumors", we have generated and used hyper-immune sera raised against certain canine recombinant mammary tumor associated proteins for the standardization of sandwich and indirect ELISA for serodiagnosis of canine mammary tumor. The sensitivity and specificities of the assay's ranges between 85-88% and 80-85%, respectively. However, an antibody against a single marker when used for different histotypes of CMT, its specificity reduced significantly. Multiplex assays are capable to detect many specific antigens in a single run whereas a traditional ELISA is used only to detect a single antigen. It has high-throughput potential, providing more results per sample, with lower sample volumes and with utmost sensitivity and specificity. Attempts are being made to increase the sensitivity and specificities of the assays by multiplexing various markers together (Fig.4).

Immunohistochemistry has been optimized using the raised polyclonal antibodies to assess tissue expression of the marker proteins in CMT (Fig.5)

We are also attempting for the development of DNA based vaccines for canine mammary tumors using certain CMT associated genes as vaccine candidates. The preclinical work including the eukaryotic expression and in vivo testing has been completed and shown promising results i.e., tumor regression after treatment with these vaccines. After efficacy treatment and finding some more vaccine candidates, these vaccines will be taken for the permission of clinical trials.

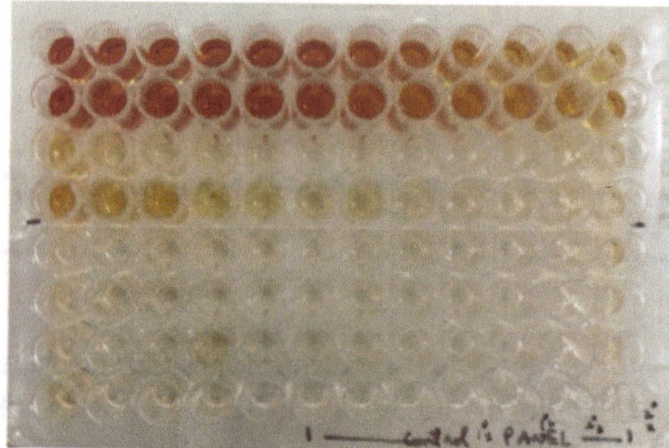

Figure 4: ELISA developed for serodiagnosis of CMT: A plate of ELISA showing different absorbances of CMT and healthy canine sera samples.

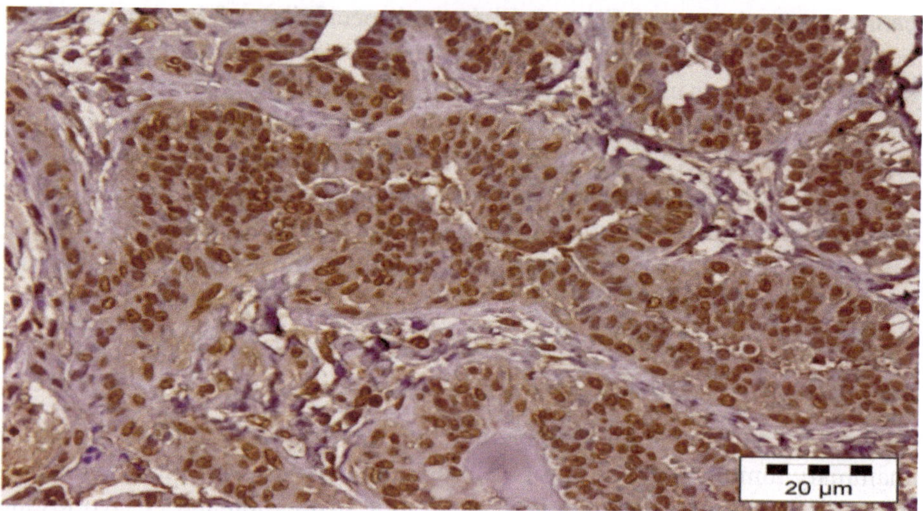

Figure 5: A representative image showing immunohistochemical profiling of CMT using the raised polyclonal antibodies against a CMT marker protein.

14

Conclusions

Mammary tumors are the most common type of neoplasia found in female dogs with high percentage of malignancy and rate of mortality. The rate of incidence of these mammary neoplasia and dysplasia is continuously advancing nationally and internationally over the last 45 years. There are different risk factors such as age, diet, hormonal exposure and breeds, which are required to be monitored in order to control the incidence of CMTs. In addition to conventional therapies such as surgical excision, radiotherapy and chemotherapy, additional precision therapeutic agents targeting TKIs, p53 tumor suppressor gene, cyclooxygenases, epithelial-mesenchymal transitions and various hormones/ hormonal receptors could be beneficial for the treatment of CMTs. Scientific efforts are also being made to develop different biomarker panels and tests for prognosis/diagnosis of the diseases as well as to develop vaccines against CMTs.

15

References

Agostini M., Enzo M. V., Bedin C., Belardinelli V., Goldin E., Del Bianco P., and Nitti D. (2012). Circulating cell-free DNA: a promising marker of regional lymphnode metastasis in breast cancer patients. Cancer Biomarkers 11 (2-3), 89-98.

Badowska-Kozakiewicz A. M., and Malicka E. (2012). Immunohistochemical evaluation of expression of heat shock proteins HSP70 and HSP90 in mammary gland neoplasms in bitches. Polish Journal of Veterinary Sciences 15 (2), 115-18.

Beffagna G., Sammarco A., Bedin C., Romualdi C., Mainenti M., MolloA. and Zappulli V. (2017). Circulating cell-free DNA in dogs with mammary tumors: short and long fragments and integrity index. PLoS One 12 (1), e0169454.

Birdi R., Kumar B. S., Gupta K., Kashyap N., & KumarA. (2019). Circulating level of heat shock protein 27 is elevated in dogs with mammary tumors. 3 Biotech 9 (6), 1-9.

Campos L. C., Lavalle G. E., Estrela-Lima A., Melgaço de Faria J. C., Guimaraes J. E., DutraA. P. and Cassali G. D. (2012). CA 15.3, CEA and LDH in dogs with malignant mammary tumors. Journal of Veterinary Internal Medicine, 26 (6), 1383-88.

Campos L. C., Silva J. O., Santos F. S., Araújo M. R., Lavalle G. E., Ferreira E., &Cassali G. D. (2015). Prognostic significance of tissue and serum HER2 and MUC1 in canine mammary cancer. Journal of Veterinary Diagnostic Investigation 27 (4), 531-35.

Carvalho M. I., Guimarães M. J., Pires I., Prada J., Silva-Carvalho R., Lopes C., &Queiroga F. L. (2013). EGFR and micro vessel density in canine malignant mammary Tumors. Research in Veterinary Science 95 (3), 1094-99.

Cayre A., Mishellany F., Lagarde N., & Penault-Llorca F. (2007). Comparison of different commercial kits for HER2 testing in breast cancer: looking for the accurate cutoff for amplification. Breast Cancer Research 9 (5), 1-10.

Conroy S. E., Sasieni P. D., Amin V., Wang D. Y., Smith P., FentimanI. S.andLatchman D. S. (1998). Antibodies to heat-shock protein 27 are associated with improved survival in patients with breast cancer. British Journal of Cancer 77 (11), 1875-79.

Dash S., Singh C. and Singh N. (2020). Studies on prevalence of mammary gland tumors of female dogs in Ludhiana, Punjab. International Journal of Livestock Research 10 (12), 235-42.

de Pedro M., Baeza S., Escudero M. T., Dierssen-Sotos T., Gómez-Acebo I., Pollán M., & Llorca J. (2015). Effect of COX-2 inhibitors and other non-steroidal inflammatory drugs on breast cancer risk: a meta-analysis. Breast Cancer Research and Treatment 149 (2), 525-36.

Dhami M.A., Tank R.H., Karle A.S., Vedpathak H.S. & Bhatia A.S. (2010). Epidemiology of canine mammary gland tumor in Gujrat. Veterinary World 3 (6): 282-85.

Di Gioia D., Blankenburg I., Nagel D., Heinemann V., & Stieber P. (2016). Tumor markers in the early detection of tumor recurrence in breast cancer patients: CA 125, CYFRA 21-1, HER2 shed antigen, LDH and CRP in combination with CEA and CA 15-3. Clinica Chimica Acta, 461, 1-7.

Garcia A. P., Reis L. A., Nunes F. C., Longford F. G., Frey J. G., de Paula A. M. and Cassali G. D. (2021). Canine mammary cancer Tumorbehaviour and patient survival time are associated with collagen fibre characteristics. Scientific Reports 11 (1), 1-13.

Gavhane D. S., Singh A., Sood N. K. and Gupta K. (2016). Expression of stem cell biomarker aldehyde dehydrogenase 1 (ALDH1) in canine mammary tumor. The Indian Journal of Animal Sciences 86 (3), 285–87.

Ghoncheh M., Pournamdar Z. and Salehiniya H. (2016). Incidence and mortality and epidemiology of breast cancer in the world. Asian Pacific Journal of Cancer Prevention 17 (sup3), 43-46.

Goldschmidt M., Peña L., Rasotto R. andZappulli V. (2011). Classification and grading of canine mammary tumors. Veterinary Pathology48 (1), 117-31.

Gray M., Meehan J., Martinez-Perez C., Kay C. and Turnbull A.K. (2020). Naturally occurring canine mammary tumors as a transitional model for human breast cancer. Frontiers in Oncology Women's Cancer. Doi= 10.3389/fonc.2020.00617.

Gupta K., Sood N.K., UppalS.K., Mohindroo J., Mahajan S., Raghunath M. and Singh K. (2012). Epidemiological Studies on Canine Mammary Tumor and its Relevance for Breast Cancer Studies. IOSR Journal of Pharmacy 2 (2): 322-33.

https://ninhealthcare.com/product/47826/the-aware-breast-self-exam-kit

https://www.cepheid.com/en/tests/Oncology-Genetics/Xpert-Breast-Cancer-STRAT4

Hugo H. J., Saunders C., Ramsay R. G. and Thompson E. W. (2015). New insights on COX-2 in chronic inflammation driving breast cancer growth and metastasis. Journal of Mammary Gland Biology and Neoplasia 20 (3), 109-19.

Hussain S., Saxena S., Shrivastava S., AroraR., Singh R. J., Jena S. C. and Singh R. K. (2018). Multiplexed autoantibody signature for serological detection of canine mammary Tumors. Scientific Reports 8 (1), 1-14.

Im K. S., Jang Y. G., Shin J. I., Kim N. H., Lim H. Y., Lee S. M.andSur J. H. (2015). CD44+/ CD24–cancer stem cells are associated with higher grade of canine mammary carcinomas. Veterinary Pathology 52 (6), 1041-44.

Jurikova M., Danihel Ľ., Polák Š.and Varga I. (2016). Ki67, PCNA, and MCM proteins: Markers of proliferation in the diagnosis of breast cancer. Acta Histochemica 118 (5), 544-52.

Kandefer-Gola M., Nowak M., Ciaputa R. and Madej J. A. (2016). Usefulness of immuno-histochemical indicators for diagnosis and prognosis of poorly differentiated Tumors. Journal of Veterinary Research 60 (3), 323-30.

Kaszak I., Ruszczak A., Kanafa S., Kacprzak K., Król M. and Jurka P. (2018). Current biomarkers of canine mammary tumors. Acta Veterinaria Scandinavica, 60 (1), 1-13.

Kato M., Yano K. I., Matsuo F., Saito H., Katagiri T., Kurumizaka H. and Miki Y. (2000). Identification of Rad51 alteration in patients with bilateral breast cancer. Journal of Human Genetics 45(3), 133-37.

Kaur N., Kumar B. V. S., Mahajan K., & Singh S. (2016). Expression and characterization of tissue inhibitor of metalloproteinase 4 from complex canine mammary carcinomas. Journal of Immunoassay and Immunochemistry 37 (5), 515-26.

Khimta S., Maiti S. K., Kumar N. and Sharma A. K. (2011). Occurrence of neoplasms in canine a retrospective study. The Indian Journal of Animal Sciences 80 (1), 7-11.

Klopfleisch R. and Gruber A. D. (2009 B). Differential expression of cell cycle regulators p21, p27 and p53 in metastasizing canine mammary adenocarcinomas versus normal mammary glands. Research in Veterinary Science 87 (1), 91-96.

Klopfleisch R. and Gruber A. D. (2009 A). Increased expression of BRCA2 and RAD51 in lymph node metastases of canine mammary adenocarcinomas. Veterinary Pathology 46 (3), 416-22.

Kumar B. S., Bhardwaj R., Mahajan K., Kashyap N., Kumar A. and Verma R. (2018). The overexpression of Hsp90B1 is associated with tumorigenesis of canine mammary glands. Molecular and Cellular Biochemistry 440 (1), 23-31.

Kumar S. B. V. and Kataria M. (2013). Identification of single nucleotide polymorphism in stromelysin-3 catalytic domain in canine mammary tumors. Journal of Applied Animal Research 41 (3), 366-69.

Kumaraguruparan R., Karunagaran D., Balachandran C., Manohar B. M. and Nagini S. (2006). Of humans and canines: a comparative evaluation of heat shock and apoptosis-associated proteins in mammary tumors. Clinicachimica acta, 365 (1-2), 168-76.

Li Z., Yin S., Zhang L., Liu W. and Chen B. (2017). Prognostic value of reduced E-cadherin expression in breast cancer: a meta-analysis. Oncotarget 8 (10), 16445-55.

Manuali E., De Giuseppe A., Feliziani F., Forti K., Casciari C., Marchesi M. C., and Król M. (2012). CA 15–3 cell lines and tissue expression in canine mammary cancer and the correlation between serum levels and Tumor histological grade. BMC Veterinary Research 8 (1), 1-10.

Miki Y., Swensen J., Shattuck-Eidens D., Futreal P. A., Harshman K., Tavtigian S. and Skolnick M. H. (1994). A strong candidate for the breast and ovarian cancer susceptibility gene BRCA1. Science 266 (5182), 66-71.

Misdorp W. (1988). Canine mammary Tumors: protective effect of late ovariectomy and stimulating effect of progestins. Veterinary Quarterly 10 (1), 26-33.

Nadhiya C., Nair M.G., Kumar R., Lakkawar A.W., Uma S. and Alphonse R.M.D. (2018). A study on the occurrence of mammary neoplasms in dogs at Puducherry, India. The Pharma Innovation Journal. 7 (7), 271-74.

Nowak, M., Madej, J. A., Pula, B., Dziegiel, P., &Ciaputa, R. (2015). Expression of matrix metalloproteinase 2 (MMP-2), E-cadherin and Ki-67 in metastatic and non-metastatic canine mammary carcinomas. Irish Veterinary Journal, 69 (1), 1-6.

Ochiai K., Morimatsu M., Tomizawa N. and Syuto B. (2001). Cloning and sequencing full length of canine Brca2 and Rad51 cDNA. Journal of Veterinary Medical Science 63(10), 1103-08.

Pan Y., Yuan Y., Liu G. and Wei Y. (2017). P53 and Ki-67 as prognostic markers in triple-negative breast cancer patients. PLoS One, 12 (2) e0172324.

Pandey M., Kumar B. S. and Verma R. (2015). Mammaglobin as a diagnostic serum marker of complex canine mammary carcinomas. Research in Veterinary Science 103, 187-92.

Pandey M., Kumar B. S., Gupta K., Sethi R. S., Kumar A. and Verma R. (2018). Over-expression of mammaglobin-B in canine mammary tumors. BMC Veterinary Research 14 (1), 1-8.

Pandey M., Kumar B. S., Singh S. and Verma R. (2017). Development of recombinant matrix metalloproteinase-3 based sandwich ELISA for sero-diagnosis of canine mammary carcinomas. Journal of Immunoassay and Immunochemistry 38 (1), 34-44.

Pandey P., Jadon N. S., Chauhan U. K., Tiwari A. K. and Singh H. (2012). Oncolytic effect of VP3 gene of chicken infectious anemia virus on canine mammary tumor cells. The Indian Journal of Animal Sciences 82 (4), 377-78.

Paoloni M. and Khanna C. (2008). Translation of new cancer treatments from pet dogs to humans. Nature Reviews Cancer 8 (2), 147-56.

Pawaiya R. S., Krishna L. and Kumar R. (2011). Genes responsible for cancer: a review. The Indian Journal of Animal Sciences 81 (8), 783-802.

Queiroga F. L., Perez-Alenza M. D., Silvan G., Peña L., Lopes C. and Illera J. C. (2005). Cox-2 levels in canine mammary tumors, including inflammatory mammary carcinoma: clinicopathological features and prognostic significance. Anticancer Research 25 (6B), 4269-75.

Queiroga F. L., Pires I., Lobo L. and Lopes C. S. (2010). The role of Cox-2 expression in the prognosis of dogs with malignant mammary Tumors. Research in Veterinary Science 88 (3), 441-45.

Queiroga F. L., Pires I., Parente M., Gregório H. and Lopes C. S. (2011 a). COX-2 over-expression correlates with VEGF and tumor angiogenesis in canine mammary cancer. The Veterinary Journal 189 (1), 77-82.

Queiroga F. L., Raposo T., Carvalho M. I., Prada J. and Pires I. (2011 b). Canine mammary Tumors as a model to study human breast cancer: most recent findings. In vivo May-June 25 (3), 455-65.

Ramaswamy S., Ross K. N., Lander E. S. and Golub T. R. (2003). A molecular signature of metastasis in primary solid tumors. Nature Genetics 33 (1), 49-54.

Ripperger T., Gadzicki D., Meindl A. and Schlegelberger B. (2009). Breast cancer susceptibility: current knowledge and implications for genetic counselling. European Journal of Human Genetics 17 (6), 722-31.

Rivera P. and Von Euler H. (2011). Molecular biological aspects on canine and human mammary tumors. Veterinary Pathology 48 (1), 132-46.

Rivera P., Melin M., Biagi T., Fall T., Häggström J., Lindblad-Toh, K. and von Euler H. (2009). Mammary tumor development in dogs is associated with BRCA1 and BRCA2. Cancer Research 69 (22), 8770-74.

Russo J. (2015). Significance of rat mammary tumors for human risk assessment. Toxicologic Pathology 43 (2), 145-70.

Savagner P P. 2010. The epithelial-mesenchymal transition (EMT) phenomenon. Annals of Oncology 21 (7): 89–92.

Saxena V., Maiti S. K., Kumar N. and Sharma A. K. (2011). Effect of cinnoline sulfonamide derivatives in canine mammary and venereal Tumors. The Indian Journal of Animal Sciences 78 (11), 59-65.

Sharma N., Gupta A.K., Bhat R.A., Yatoo M.I. and Parray O.R. (2018). Epidemiology and treatment of canine mammary tumors in Jammu region of India. Journal of Dairy Veterinary and Animal Research 7 (2), 59-62.

Sonnenschein E. G., Glickman L. T., Goldschmidt M. H. and McKee L. J. (1991). Body conformation, diet, and risk of breast cancer in pet dogs: a case-control study. American Journal of Epidemiology 133 (7), 694-703.

Sorenmo K. U., Kristiansen V. M, Comfone M. A., Shofer F. S., Breen A. M., Langeland M., Mongil C. M., Grondahl A. M., Teige J. and Goldschmidt M.H. (2010). Canine mammary gland tumors; a histological continuum from benign to malignant; clinical and histopathological evidence. Veterinary Comparative Oncology 7 (3), 162–72.

Tabaran A. and Toma G.C. (2016). The dog–a genetic model for the spontaneous tumors. Revista Romana de MedicinaVeterinara 26 (3), 15-21.

Torre L. A., Bray F., Siegel R. L., Ferlay J., Lortet-Tieulent J. and Jemal A. (2015). Global cancer statistics, 2012. CA: A cancer Journal for Clinicians 65 (2), 87-108.

Umeshwori N., Kumar A., Tyagi S. P. and Kurade N. P. (2011). Incidence and management of neoplasms in dogs of Himachal Pradesh. The Indian Journal of Animal Sciences 81 (1), 26-28.

Verma A. K., Jadon N. S., Pandey P. and Tiwari A. K. (2014). Gross, histopathological and electron microscopic studies of canine mammary gland tumor treated with NS1 gene of canine parvo virus. The Indian Journal of Animal Sciences 84 (4), 373-78.

Walsh T., Casadei S., Coats K. H., Swisher E., Stray S. M., Higgins J. and King M. C. (2006). Spectrum of mutations in BRCA1, BRCA2, CHEK2, and TP53 in families at high risk of breast cancer. Journal of American Medical Association 295 (12), 1379-88.

Wooster R., Neuhausen S. L., Mangion J., Quirk Y., Ford D., Collins N. and Stratton M. R. (1994). Localization of a breast cancer susceptibility gene, BRCA2, to chromosome 13q12-13. Science 265 (5181), 2088-90.

Zajkowska M., Głażewska E. K., Będkowska G. E., Chorąży P., Szmitkowski M. and Ławicki S. (2016). Diagnostic power of vascular endothelial growth factor and macrophage colony-stimulating factor in breast cancer patients based on ROC analysis. Mediators of Inflammation 2016 Article ID 5962946 | https://doi.org/10.1155/2016/5962946.

16

Index

A
Adenocarcinomas 3, 7
Adenomas 7
ALDH1 17, 18
Anaplastic carcinomas 7

B
Babesiosis 1
Bcl 17, 21, 23
Benign tumors 3, 5
Biomarkers 17, , 29, 30, 31
BRCA 31

C
Canine 1, 2, 5, 7, 8, 9, 10, 11, 12, 13, 17, 19, 19, 22, 23, 24, 27, 29, 30, 32, 33, 34
Canine distemper 1
Canine Mammary Tumors 1, , 5, 7, 8, 13, 17, 19, 29, 32, 33
Canine parvoviral diarrhoea 1
Carcinogenesis 10, 25
CHEK2 15
Classification and Grading 7
Companion animals 1, 9
COX inhibitors 21, 26
Cyclooxygenases 23, 26, 35

D
Deracoxib 21, 26
Diagnosis 19, 20
Doxorubicin 21

E
EMT 17, 25
Epidemiology 11
Estrogen receptors 20
FGFR2 15

F
Fibroadenomas 7

G
GADVASU 33

H
Haemoprotozoans 1
HER-2 20, 24, 26, 27, 29, 30, 31, 32
Histopathology 11
Hormones 9, 13, 14, 15, 23, 35
HSP 16, 32
Human breast cancer 9, 15, 20, 23

I
Immunohistochemistry 16, 20
Incidence 2, 11, 12, 13, 14, 15, 35
Infectious canine hepatitis 1

K
Kennel cough 1
Ki-67 17, 20, 30

L
Leptospirosis 1
Leukemia 21

M
Malignant tumors 5, 7, 1121, 29, 31
Mammary Tumors 1, 2, 3, 5, 7, 8, 11, 13, 13, 14, 15, 17, 19, 21, 22, 26, 27, 29, 30, 32, 33, 35
MAP3K1 15
Metastasis 3, 7, 8, 16, 19, 23, 25, 30
Mucin-1 27, 29
Myoepithelial cells 8, 19

N

Neoplasm 2, 9, 17
NSAID 22, 29

O

Obesity 1, 2, 3, 14
Oncogenes 15, 17
Ovariohysterectomy 23

P

PCNA 17, 29, 30
PDGFR 25
Piroxicam 22
Predisposing Factors 1, 13
Prevalence 2, 9, 11
Progesterone receptors 20
Prognosis 3, 7, 17, 21, 22, 29, 30, 31, 33, 35
PTEN 15

R

Rabies 1
RAD51 15, 16
RAS 17

S

SERMS 23
Skin neoplasia 2
Solid carcinomas 7

T

Treatment 1, 3, 7, 19, 20, 21, 22, 23, 24, 25, 29, 33, 35
Tubular adenocarcinomas 7
TUNEL assay 24
Tyro-kinase inhibitors 24

V

Vaccination 1
VEGFR 25

W

World Health Organization 7